Yoga For Beginners

A simple guide to a slim body, stress relief and inner peace

Nicole Talbot

Credits – All photos;

Photography by: Barney Douglas as www.bdfoto.co.uk

Model: Charlotte Benn

ISBN: 1512296643
ISBN-13: 978-1512296648

Introduction

I want to thank you and congratulate you for downloading the book, *"Yoga For Beginners"*.

This book contains proven steps and strategies on how to perform many yoga postures and techniques at home with no prior experience.

It provides a brief outline of the styles of yoga, the chakra system and the various teaching approaches. The beginner will be guided through ways to choose a class or style to match their goals and personality. The book also provides helpful tips on getting started and mistakes to avoid.

There are sections devoted to weight loss, stress relief, attaining inner peace, easy morning routines and classic postures. Each posture is described in detail with an accompanying image and a list of related physical, mental and emotional benefits.

Contents

What's in this book?

You've opened this book because you are curious about the nature of yoga and how it can benefit you. At the same time you may be a little hesitant as you think it might be 'too spiritual' or that you are not flexible enough. Or maybe you see yoga as just a lot of poses that don't really give you a proper workout.

While it's true that yoga has a deep spiritual history and focus, this book will focus on the physical asanas, or postures, that you can use every day. You will see how you can use these asanas to improve your body in many ways including weight loss, toned muscles, stress relief, boosted immunity, improved concentration and inner calm. You will also gain lots of tips for getting yourself started.

The book can be read from start to finish or you can simply pick out the chapters that interest you most. Use it as your own self-paced guide or for daily practice between classes.

Everyone can 'do' yoga; it's just a matter of finding the approach that suits your nature and ability. Remember to go at your own pace, there is no competition or goals to score and fastest is not always best. It is all about self-improvement and learning to take charge of your body. So take a deep breath and enjoy the process.

Chapter 1

What is yoga?

The term 'yoga' means 'union' or to be more specific – the union of the individual soul with the universal soul. It encompasses the journey that individuals must take in order to transcend the self and become part of the whole. It is not a religious practice but its themes align with the goals of many religions i.e.; to become one with God/Allah/the universe.

Its origins can be traced back many centuries in India where all the knowledge was documented in Sanskrit meaning that only the elite could read and practice it. The ancient yogis recognized that people learn in different ways so the six pathways to union were developed.

These are:

- Jinana – union through knowledge/intellect
- Bhakti – union through devotion
- Karma – union through action
- Mantra – union through sound/incantations
- Hatha – union through bodily control
- Raja – union through mental control

Yoga has since spread across the globe and is practiced using many combinations of these pathways.

In India, the practice remains close to its traditional roots and many people embrace the full range of yoga disciplines as part of their daily lives. Western society, however, is generally more focused on the physical benefits of Hatha yoga and to a lesser extent, Raja yoga.

What are chakras?

The ancient yogis believed that the body contains seven centers of energy or 'chakras'. These are positioned vertically from the base of the spine to the crown of the head. Each is associated with a particular set of internal bodily functions and external influences and also with a specific color. The chakras can be viewed as a place where we send and receive energy. They can be blocked by emotions and limiting beliefs which can create an imbalance in the energy associated with that chakra.

- **Muladhara or Root Chakra**

  The color for this chakra is red and it is located around the base of the spine. The root chakra energy is focused around being connected to the earth or feeling grounded, feeling safe and secure, being calm and composed and also with removing waste from the body. It encompasses the lower limbs and the large intestine and stimulates the gonads.

- **Svadisthana Chakra**

  The second chakra is orange and it is located behind and just below the navel. It involves the hips and lower areas of the torso including the hips, reproductive organs, bladder and kidneys. Svadisthana is associated with emotions, sexuality, sensuality and intimacy.

- **Manipura Chakra**

  The energy of Manipura Chakra is associated with our vitality, trust, relationships, self-esteem, digestion and adaptability. Its color is yellow and it is located in our solar plexus area above the naval. This chakra radiates energy though all the internal organs including the pancreas where it helps to regulate blood sugar.

- **Anahata Chakra**

  The fourth chakra is known as the Heart Chakra and it relates to love and breath. It is the crossover point between the lower chakras that focus on our physical energies and the upper chakras that deal with our spiritual energies. Its color is green and it includes the upper chest and back.

This chakra helps to regulate the immune system though the thymus gland.

- **Visuddha Chakra**

  This chakra is centered in the areas around the neck, jaw and throat working on the thyroid and parathyroid glands. Its color is turquoise blue and the energy focus is spiritual. It is associated with our inner 'voice' and communication in all forms.

- **Ajna Chakra**

  This chakra is often referred to as the 'third eye' as it is located in the centre of the forehead. It is concerned with how we 'see' outside the realms of the physical world. The energy of this chakra is focused on visualization, intuition, dreaming, and also telepathy. Its color is indigo and it relates to the pineal gland.

- **Sahasrara Chakra**

  The seventh chakra is associated with violet and it is positioned at the crown of the head regulating the pituitary gland. It is the chakra concerned with the energy of thought, enlightenment and our beliefs. It controls our highest mental and spiritual functions.

Types of yoga

There are many types or schools of yoga. Some are centuries old while others have been developed over the last few decades. The most common types include:

- **Hatha**

  This is a broad genre encompassing a series of gentle, slow-paced postures and relaxation.

- **Vinyassa**

  This more vigorous form uses breath-synchronized postures.

- **Astingar**

  In this fast paced form the focus is on constant, flowing movement through a series of postures.

- **Iyengar**

  Here the focus is on alignment and holding postures while paused in full stretch. It uses many props such as yoga bricks and belts to help pull the body into alignment.

- **Bikram**

  This is performed in a room heated to around 100 degrees. The heat relaxes the muscles and the sweat releases toxins from the body.

The postures in this book are based on a *Hatha style* approach.

Chapter 2

What are your goals?

To lose weight?

While all forms of yoga will help you burn calories, the more physically challenging ones such as Bikram and Ashtanga can be just as effective as an intensive gym work out.

Once you have been practicing yoga regularly you will also notice that you are more conscious of your body's needs. You will start to gravitate towards healthier food choices and may start to notice the flavor of your food as you eat more slowly.

Stress is one of the biggest causes of over-eating so as you become calmer overall you may find that you no longer have as many cravings for comfort food.

To decrease stress?

Stress generally comes from external factors such as relationships and careers. When we get stressed our bodies can hold a lot of tension in the muscles and our breathing gets restricted. Yoga works on the whole body and can focus on the trouble spots full of knots and dissipate them. Slower breathing and a quiet environment promote a sense of calm. The mind has time to reflect and to allow any stressful thoughts to come to the surface to be recognized and then dismissed.

To promote calm?

The practice of yoga generates a sense of 'wholeness' and peace within us. It teaches us not only see the details but also the bigger picture so we see things in perspective. It keeps us grounded.

Emotional blockages can build up tension in our bodies over time. Postures that target these tension spots can help release the pent up emotion that caused them.

Choosing a class or style

Try and choose a class or style that matches your personality. Do you prefer to exercise alone or in a group with an instructor? Would you like your session to be slow or fast paced?

It is a good idea to try out a few different classes and styles to find your best fit. If you want to attend a class then being in a pleasant environment and having a good connection with the instructor is vital. You need to be able to ask for help and also to say 'no' if something doesn't feel right. Above all, you need to enjoy the whole experience.

Your level of fitness and experience will play a part. A beginner should not attempt an advanced class or advanced postures as they may cause injury to themselves or be discouraged from going further as it was too hard.

Getting started

Wear loose, comfortable clothing that you don't mind sweating in. Avoid clothing with zips, buckles or buttons especially over the abdominal area. Be aware that you may be in an inverted position so avoid clothing that will come loose and cause you embarrassment. Yoga is best done in bare feet but socks are fine providing you don't slip in them.

Most Hatha yoga postures need no props and can be done anywhere, however you may want to use a yoga mat for grip and comfort. If you are on a timber or tiled floor a carpet or rug is fine. Many balance postures can be performed up against a wall initially until you gain strength and confidence.

If you suffer from hip, knee or back problems, you may find that sitting on a rolled up towel or placing it under your joints may ease the pressure on them in some postures. Yoga bricks or blocks can serve the same purpose. These are especially useful in postures such as the Child's pose or the Corpse pose. If you have trouble reaching your feet in postures such as the Seated Forward Bend you could loop a belt or tie around your feet and pull against that.

Many postures can also be modified and performed sitting in a chair or holding one for support and balance. Some can even be performed while lying in bed. Experiment and find what works best for you. Some yoga studios run chair-based yoga classes for those with arthritis or other physical limitations.

Most yoga routines follow the same basic sequence. They begin with some breathing exercises then warm up stretches such as the Salute to the Sun (which we will cover later in this book). They then continue through a series starting with the standing postures to release and strengthen the body. Next comes the sitting and twisting postures for deeper stretches and then the inverted postures for cleansing the body and reversing the blood flow. Finally the sessions finish with some relaxation and breathing postures to wind down.

Many yoga classes end with a simple meditation session. A warm blanket and low pillow may help you become more comfortable while lying on your back and ease you into a relaxed state of mind.

To create your optimal environment for practicing yoga, remove any external distractions. Turn off the TV, put your phone on silent and have someone else look after the kids. If you want to you can put on any music that you find peaceful and soothing or you may prefer total quiet. In a class environment, allow space between yourself and the next person and try to tune out from any external noise.

Precautions

If you have a medical condition that you think may be affected by practicing yoga such as neck, back or blood pressure issues, be sure to seek the advice of a qualified instructor and also your doctor beforehand.

Pregnant women should also seek advice first. Some postures may be dangerous for the baby or cause you discomfort. Pre-natal yoga classes are a better alternative.

Women who are menstruating can experience low energy levels so it is best to stick to gentle postures that don't overheat the body. Avoid the inverted postures that raise the hips such as the shoulder stand and replace them with inverted leg postures that don't raise the hips. You can also try seated postures that open out the hips and pelvic area. These can also help to relieve cramps.

Never do a yoga session after a big meal as this may cause you discomfort when using the abdominal muscles or lying on the floor face down. A full stomach can also lower your energy. Also avoid practicing yoga late at night as its stimulating effect may keep you awake. The exception to this is when you choose calming postures or mental relaxation exercises to encourage sleep.

Beginner's tips

When you are starting out it is tempting to want to do each posture perfectly, but as with anything else, perfection takes regular practice. Take it at your own pace and don't compete with yourself or anyone else. There are no winners or losers. Be wary of going straight into the postures. Always do some gentle warm up stretches first.

"No pain, no gain" does not really apply in yoga. While it is normal to feel some discomfort when stretching your body beyond its comfort zone, pushing too far past your limits may cause injury. It may feel at first as though gentle movements are not helping you at all but after some regular practice you will soon start to see the benefits so be patient and progress steadily. It is also normal to experience surges of emotion in some postures. This is a natural release of energy and is no cause for concern.

When you begin practicing yoga you may find that it can be difficult to keep your mind focused inwards. Each posture works on different aspects of the body and it is beneficial to focus on that aspect as you perform the posture. For example, the Cobra or Bhujangasana works on the heart and the thymus gland which aids the immune system.

If you are not sure exactly what the posture does you can still focus on how your muscles, tendons and joints move while in that posture. You may even be able to visualize the flow of blood, oxygen and energy moving through your body.

To begin with, hold your postures for up to a minute but remember to breathe. Many beginners tense up while holding the postures and hold their breath. Use the breath to your advantage. Breathe in gently and use your exhalations to help extend your stretch a little further each time.

Use your diaphragm to control your breath. Try lying on your back and placing your hands on either side of the diaphragm. Breathe in slowly and feel the air expanding under your lower ribs and into your sides and lower back. Feel your hands rising and falling gently.

Focus on alignment. Yoga is very much about creating balance both internally and externally. When you do a posture that stretches your left side, repeat it on the right. Also, follow a forward bend with a backward one and vice versa. You may find that one side is stiffer than the other and that's normal, just be sure to devote the same amount of energy to each side even if the results may differ. Yoga also helps to balance the left and right sides of the brain.

Maintaining correct spinal alignment is particularly important in preventing injury and improving posture. To check your alignment, stand barefoot with your back against a wall. Place your feet directly under your hips and have your shoulders touch the wall. Notice the position of your lower back and abdomen. Are they in line with your hips and shoulders or are they pushed out in front? If they are sitting forward, then tighten your abdominal muscles and pull them towards the wall, tilting your hips forward as you do so.

It also helps to imagine that you have a string attached to the crown of your head and someone is pulling it up. Feel the rest of your body automatically straighten up and your diaphragm expand.

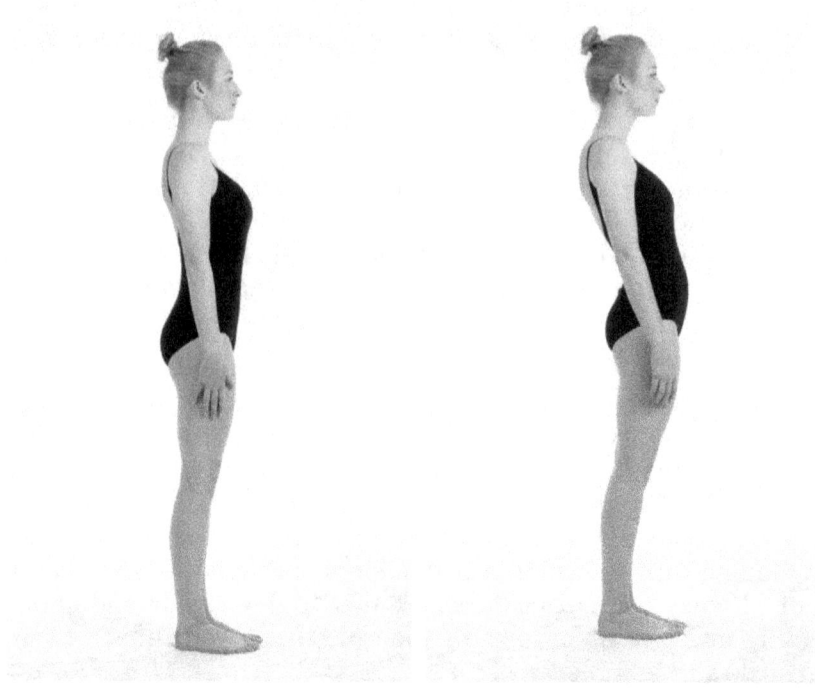

Good Posture   **Bad Posture**

Many postures begin with a neutral standing pose called the Mountain pose or Tadasana. In this pose the feet are together and the body weight is distributed evenly over both feet. Aim to maintain awareness of your posture in all standing poses (and in your everyday life).

Whenever a posture involves a straight stretch of the spine, keep the following points in mind: roll your pelvis forward towards the naval, push the tailbone down, extend the neck and pull up from the crown. Always try to keep the shoulders rolled back and down to open out the chest area and avoid hunching.

Keep your feet flat and heels on the floor unless otherwise specified. Use the floor for resistance and push against it as needed. A good example of this is the Downward Facing Dog pose.

If you are doing a series of postures it is usually advisable to have a short rest in between each one. This allows the heart rate to settle and the body to store energy for future use, rather like having our own internal charger.

These pauses can be done in several ways. From a standing position, simply drop forward and allow the head, torso and arms to hang freely from the waist or you could just drop the head to the chest and relax the neck. If your back is sore you could bend the knees and drop into a squat, allowing the pelvis to curl forward. From a sitting position, hug the knees to the chest and rest your forehead on your knees. You can also try lifting both feet off the ground and balance on your sitting bones.

If you are lying on your stomach, bring your arms alongside your body, turn your head to one side and rest your ear on the floor. To rest between postures while lying on your back, hug your knees to your chest and hold them there for a moment or move into Corpse pose.

Chapter 3

Yoga for weight loss

Health and fitness magazines and websites are loaded with marketing telling us the latest way to lose weight. 'Try this diet", "Sign up for gym membership", "Go on a weekend boot camp". While many of these are genuine and proven they imply that you need to go somewhere or spend money before you can start to lose weight. Some can also imply that being thin equates to being beautiful.

Yoga can be practiced almost anywhere at any time. All you need is a small space around you, the details of a few simple postures and the desire to get moving.

It doesn't matter what size or shape you are, yoga will help you to burn calories and tone your body. You may not see instant results but you will notice a difference as you progress. The style of yoga you choose will also influence your rate of weight loss. (Refer to the styles mentioned earlier in this book).

Yoga teachings encourage acceptance and non-discrimination so you will never be judged on your appearance or ability. Some people are naturally curvaceous so instead of aiming to be as skinny as a supermodel, it is healthier to focus on strengthening the whole body and improving the efficiency of the internal systems.

We gain weight for all sorts of reasons including genetic factors, medications, restricted mobility, lack of motivation and poor diet. Some of these are within our control and some are not.

We often create excuses for not exercising such as not having enough time, money or the right equipment. Many people are not aware that they can lose weight through practicing yoga regularly. It takes as little as 5 minutes a day although 30 – 60 minutes is more preferable. You can pick the postures that suit you and do them in your lounge room each morning. The "Salute to the Sun" outlined in Chapter 6 is a full body workout that is perfect for busy people.

Here are some postures that will get those calories burning. Hold each pose for as long as you feel comfortable and breathe into it, extending the stretch with each exhalation. Remember to do some warm up and warm down stretches as well to avoid injury.

Side Reclining Leg Lift – Anantasana

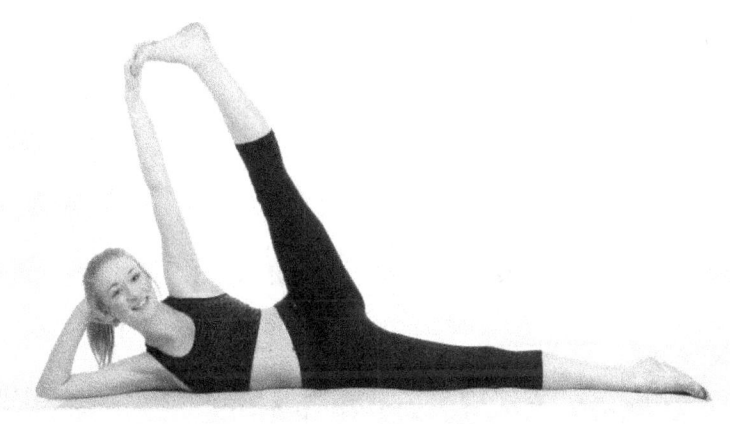

Description:

Starting Position

Lie on your right side with your right arm bent and your head resting on your hand.

Step 1

Turn the toes of your left leg towards the ceiling, bend the left knee and bring it towards the body.

Step 2

Use your left hand and grab the left big toe. Take a deep breath and when you exhale, straighten the left leg so the sole of the foot is towards the ceiling with the heel extended. Try to avoid leaning the left leg to the back or front. Pull the left leg towards the head to create the stretch.

Step 3

Hold the stretch, then keeping your grip on the toe, bend the left knee and bring the left foot down. Release your grip and straighten the left leg out. Roll over into Corpse pose and relax. Repeat on your opposite side.

Chakra: Svadisthana

Benefits:

- Reduced fat on the sides of the torso
- More flexible hips
- Firmer and stronger abdominal and leg muscles
- Improved menstrual and menopausal symptoms
- Increased sexuality and sensuality

Extended Triangle - Utthita Trikonasana

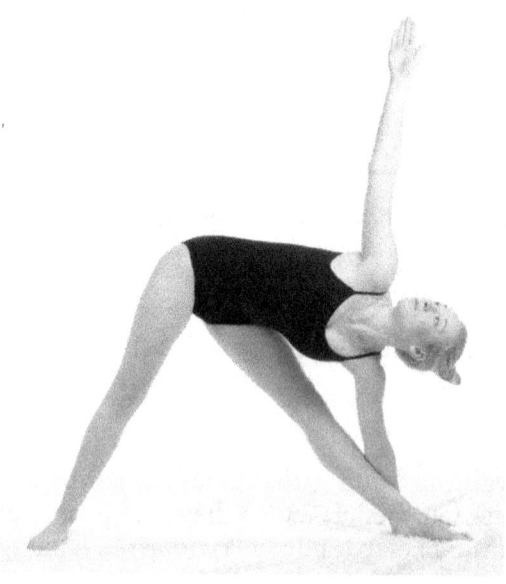

Description:

Starting Position

Begin in Mountain pose then jump or step your legs roughly 4 feet apart.

Step 1

Remain facing the front and extend both arms out to the sides as far as you can with the palms facing downwards. Aim to keep your arms in a horizontal line.

Step 2

Rotate the toes of your left foot a little towards the right. Turn the toes of the right foot to the right by 90 degrees.

Step 3

Turn your head to the right and watch the fingers as you exhale and lower the right arm to the floor beside your ankle. If you can't reach the floor, rest your right hand on the right leg as far down as you can. Bend from the hip joint rather than the waist.

Step 4

Check that your left arm is still pointing upwards and in line with the right. Once you are balanced, turn your head and look up at your left hand. Hold.

Step 5

When you are ready, slowly turn your head and look down at your right hand. Keeping both arms stretched out and your spine straight tilt yourself back into a standing position. Watch your right arm as it comes up.

Step 6

Turn your head and then your toes to the front, gently lower your arms to your sides and step your feet together. Pause and rest for a moment in Mountain pose. Repeat on your opposite side.

Chakra: Svadisthana and Manipura

Benefits:

- Tighter and stronger muscles from the feet to the neck
- Improved posture
- Improved flexibility and strength in ankles, knees, hips, spine and shoulders
- Improved digestion and metabolism
- Reduced pain from sciatica, tight neck and backaches
- Reduced stress and anxiety
- Reduced symptoms of infertility, menopause and menstruation

*Skull Shining Breath - **Kapalabhati Pranayama***

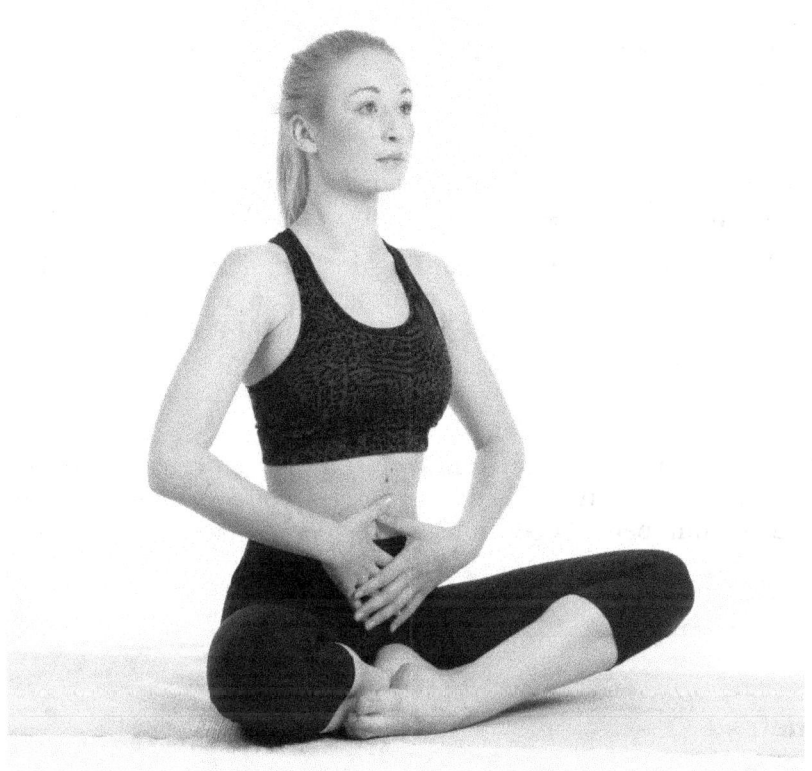

Description:

This oddly named posture is a breathing exercise (or pranayama) that focuses on flushing out or 'brightening' the inner lining of the skull and sending oxygen through the body. The Sanskrit word 'Bhati' means 'light' and refers to perception, knowledge and intelligence.

Starting Position

Begin by sitting in a comfortable, cross-legged position with the back straight.

Step 1

Place your hands together over the lower abdomen between the naval and the pubis and keep your mind focused on this area.

Step 2

Inhale slowly and feel your lower abdomen expand into your hands.

Step 3

To help you learn to isolate the lower abdominal muscles use your hands to physically push the air out of your body.

Rapidly exhale while pushing against the lower abdominal muscles. As you inhale again your abdomen will automatically relax. As you get use to this technique you should start with slower breaths – roughly one full breath cycle per second.

Step 4

Repeat the process 10 times and then relax. When you start to gain more control of your abdominal muscles you can increase your speed and number of repetitions to 25, 50 and then 100 or more.

Chakra: Manipura

Benefits:

- Improved digestion and metabolism
- Stronger and tighter abdominal muscles
- Weight loss
- Increased energy
- Improved assertiveness and determination

Warrior Pose 1 - Virabhadrasana I

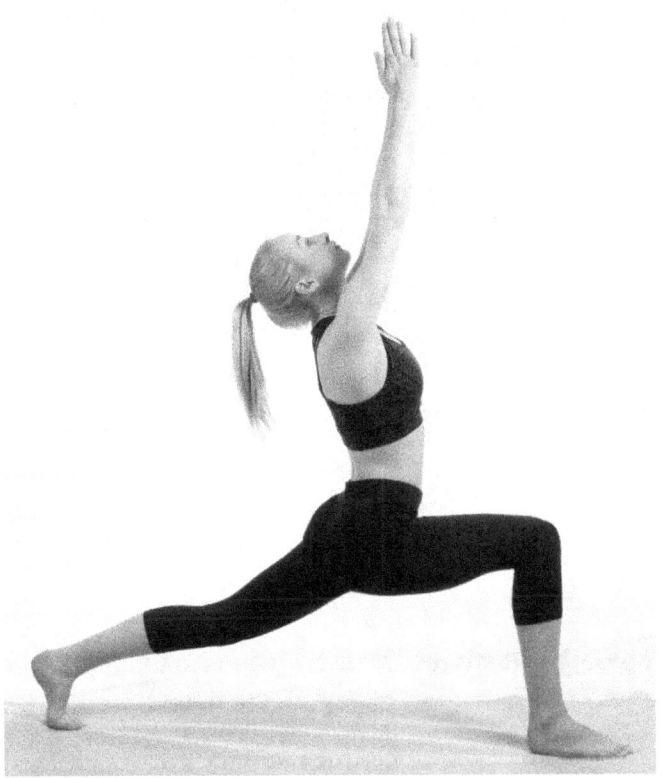

Description:

Starting Position

Stand in the Mountain pose and then lightly jump your feet apart about 3-4 feet.

Step 1

Raise your arms to the ceiling and reach up through the little fingers.

Step 2

Rotate the toes of your left foot a little towards the right. Turn the toes of the right foot to the right by 90 degrees.

Step 3
With your hands still raised, exhale and swing your hips around so your head and torso face the right.

Step 4
Exhale and lunge your right knee over your right ankle keeping your shin at a 90 degree angle to the floor.

Step 5
Stretch your body in a backwards arch and lift your chest up and away from your pelvis while you hold the pose. You should feel this stretch through your whole body.

Step 6
Release by stretching up through the arms and straightening the right knee. Turn the head and torso to the front followed by the toes. Stretch your arms out to the sides then slowly lower them to your body.

Repeat on your opposite side then return to Mountain pose.

Chakra: Muladhara, Svadisthana, Manipura and Anahata

Benefits:

- Stronger and firmer muscles throughout the body from top to bottom
- Reduced sciatica
- Improved lung capacity
- Multiple emotional and mental benefits through the stimulation of the first four chakras

Boat Pose – Paripurna Navasana

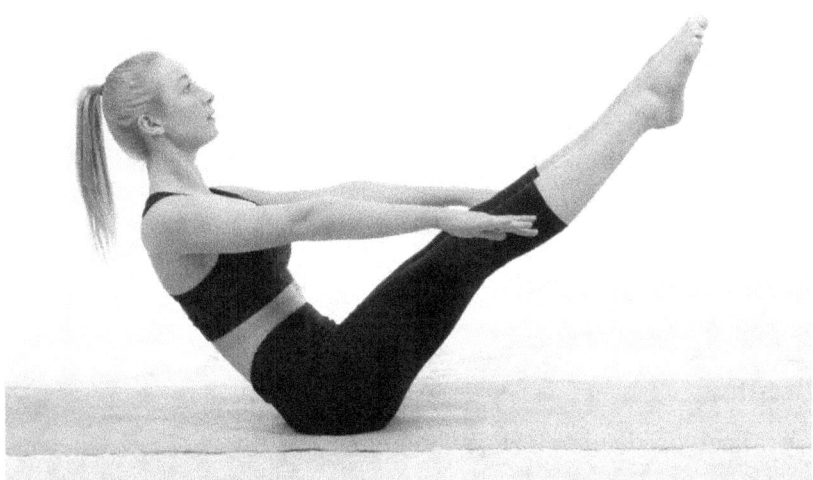

Description:

Starting Position

Sit on the floor with your back upright and your legs together straight out in front of you.

Step 1

Place your palms flat on the floor just behind the hips. Lean back slightly and position your weight evenly over your tailbone and sitting bones, tightening the buttocks.

Step 2

Breathe in then on the exhalation draw both knees up towards the chest and lift the feet up so that the thighs are at about a 45 degree angle to the floor.

Step 3

Keep your weight balanced on your buttocks. Raise your arms parallel to the floor with straight elbows and palms facing down.

Step 4

Using your core muscles for support, raise your feet and straighten your legs as much as possible with your toes flexed. If you find this difficult, try keeping your knees bent, keeping your hands on the floor or place them around the back of the thighs. Hold.

Step 5

Slowly release by lowering the feet and rolling forward into a cross-legged position. Repeat three times then lie back and rest in Corpse pose.

Chakra: Manipura

Benefits:

- Increased core strength and energy
- Tighter abdomen and buttocks
- Improved function of kidneys, digestion, thyroid and prostate glands
- Reduced stress
- Improved willpower

Chapter 4

Yoga for stress relief

Stress is part of life. There is good and bad stress. Good stress could include the butterflies you get before a presentation or performance. It helps drive us to achieve our goals and find solutions to problems. Bad stress is when we start to feel physically tense or ill in adverse situations.

Common causes of stress include relationships, deadlines, finance, illness or concern for the future.

Often it is not the situation itself that causes stress but rather it is how we interpret and react to that situation. In many cases we also believe that our stress is caused by external factors such as our work environment or a particular person.

When we experience stress over an extended period it can start to affect the body. Our muscles tense up, our blood pressure increases and we tend to take shallower, rapid breaths. Over time this creates knots in the muscles which can get tighter and tighter especially in the back, shoulders, chest and thighs. Shorter breaths don't bring as much oxygen into the body so our organs can suffer. It is well documented that prolonged stress can lead to illness in various forms.

Stress can also affect our mental state often making us anxious, forgetful or giving us a sense of 'brain fog'. We may find it hard to see past the immediate issues and gain perspective on the bigger picture. Also, when we get very tired or frazzled we often reach for sugary foods and drinks to get a quick energy boost. These then contribute to the problem.

Yoga can relieve stress by lowering blood pressure, focusing on balance within the body and using deep stretches to release tension. Regular practice builds up a reserve store of energy that helps sustain us in our everyday lives naturally. Focusing on our breathing increases our concentration and helps us to develop clarity in our thinking.

The seven chakras or energy centers are focus points for our various emotions. If we are experiencing strong negative emotions such as fear, anger or anxiety it means that corresponding chakra is blocked or overloaded. By doing postures specifically related to that chakra we allow the body to release the negative energy and bring the emotions back into balance.

The following postures are helpful in managing stress levels.

Standing Forward Bend - Uttanasana

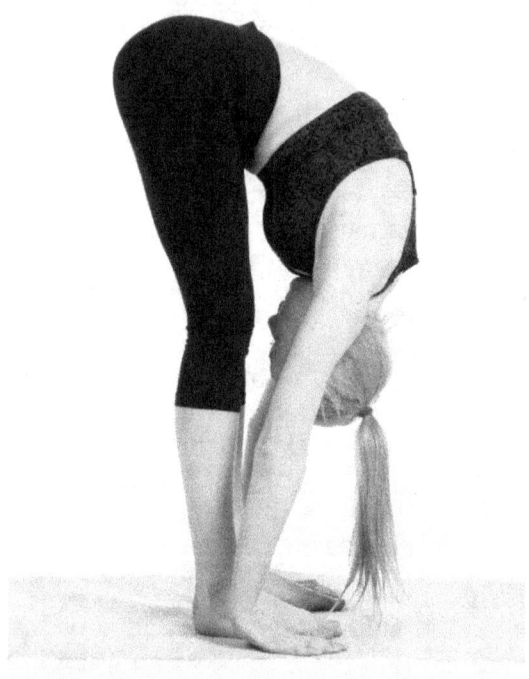

Description:

This pose can be used to relieve a stiff or sore back anytime or as a counter-posture to any backward bending pose.

Starting Position

Stand in the Mountain pose with your hands on your hips.

Step 1

Take a deep breath and as you exhale bend forward with a straight back and slide your hands down your legs as far as you can. If possible, place your hands on the floor or hold the back of your ankles or calves. Alternatively, release your hold on the legs and cross your forearms to hold the opposite elbow letting your arms drop loosely.

Step 2

With each exhalation increase your stretch and lift your tailbone upwards. Allow your head to hang loose while elongating your neck. Hold.

Step 3

To release the pose place your hands on your hips, come up with a straight back and pivot the tailbone down to return to Mountain pose. Repeat three times then rest.

Chakra: Muladhara

Benefits:

- Reduced lower back pain
- Improved ability to slow down and remain calm
- Increased sense of security and safety
- Improved flexibility in hips, quadriceps and hamstrings

Chair Pose – Utkatasana

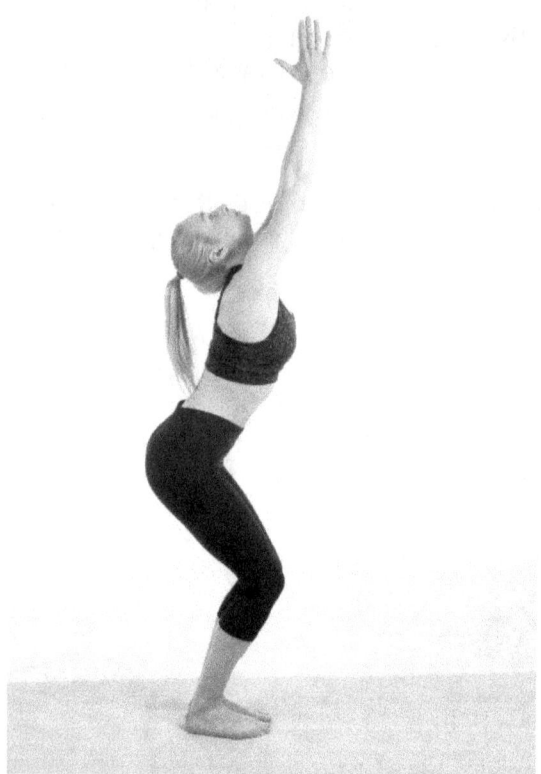

Description:

Starting Position

Begin in Mountain pose.

Step 1

Raise your arms to the ceiling. Your palms can either be touching in Prayer pose or just facing inwards without touching.

Step 2

Breathe out and slowly bend your knees keeping them aligned and the feet facing forward. As you deepen into the squat, your torso will lean forward at an angle to your thighs. Continue to lower your tailbone down towards your heels on each exhalation. Hold.

Step 3

To release the pose slowly straighten your knees while you reach to the ceiling. Exhale and bring your arms back to your sides. Repeat three times then rest.

Chakra: Muladhara and Svadisthana

Benefits:

- Improved strength in calves, thighs, ankles and feet
- Increased flexibility in spine and reduced back pain
- Increased passion and desire
- Reduced tension in thighs, abdomen, shoulders and chest
- Increased sense of calm and more open diaphragm

Cat / Cow Pose – Chakravakasana

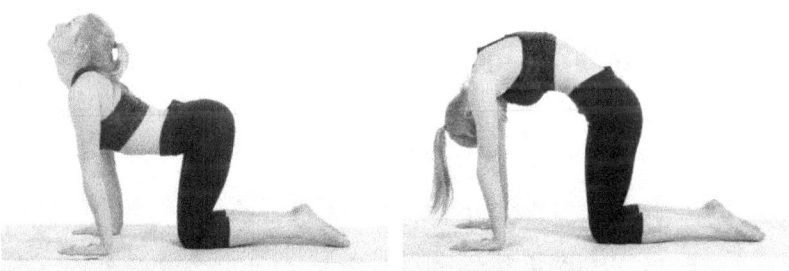

Description:

This is actually a combination of two poses – the Cat (Marjariasana) and the Cow (Bitilasana). Each is a counter pose to the other.

Starting Position

Start on your hands and knees with your wrists under your shoulders and your knees under your hips. Face the floor.

Step 1

Begin the backbend (Cow pose) by swinging the tailbone up to the ceiling and pushing your naval towards the floor. Raise your chin and look up at the ceiling. Extend the stretch from your chin through the torso to your hips and hold.

Step 2

Exhale and return to a neutral position.

Step 3

Move into the Cat pose by tightening your abdominal muscles, rotating the tailbone and hips forward then hunching your back up towards the ceiling. Slowly curl your neck forward with the crown of the head towards the floor and look towards your pelvis and hold.

Step 4

You can move between the two postures in one fluid motion. Inhale in the Cow pose and exhale in the Cat pose, using the hips and abdomen to control the movement and letting the neck and head follow. Continue for several breaths then return the spine to the neutral position. Sit back on your heels and rest in Child's pose.

Chakra: Svadisthana, Manipura and Anahata

Benefits:

- Improved core strength and posture
- Reduced tension and pain in lower back
- Firmer muscles across the front of the chest and neck
- Reduced stress and body tension
- Improved supply of oxygen through the blood stream
- Reduced symptoms of menstruation and menopause
- Increased sense of balance and harmony in the mind and body

Cow Faced Pose – Gomukhasana

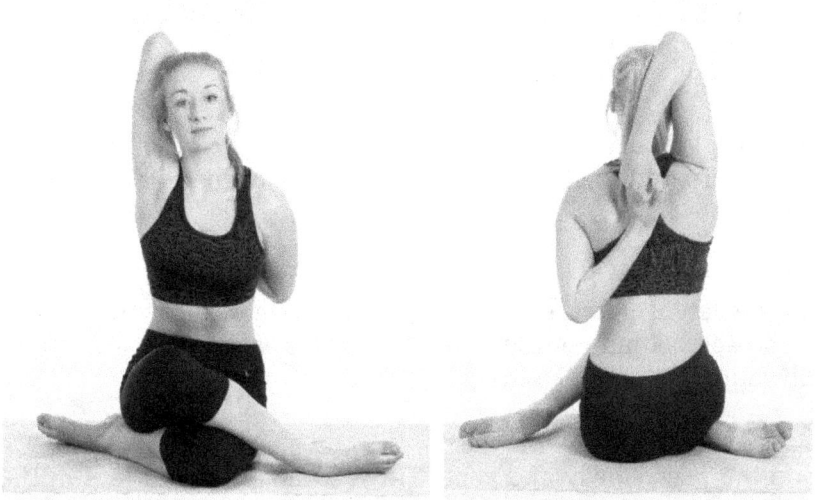

Description:

Starting Position

Sit up with your feet out straight in front of you

Step 1

Bend your knees up so your feet are flat on the floor.

Step 2

Push your left foot under the right knee. Lower the left knee to the floor. Sit evenly over the sitting bones.

Step 3

Raise the right leg and lift it over the left leg so that the right knee rests on top of the left knee. Push the heels towards the opposite hips.

Alternatively, you can simply sit in a comfortable cross-legged position.

Step 4

Stretch the right arm to the side and swing it around behind you with the palm up. Press this arm into the lower back with the back of the hand against the spine. Gradually work the forearm upwards and aim to place it parallel to the spine. Reach up as far as you can and hold.

Step 5

Take your left arm and point it straight out in front of you. Turn the palm up and raise your arm towards the ceiling lifting as high as you can.

Step 6

Bend the left arm and keep the elbow pointing towards the ceiling. Reach back behind your left shoulder as far as you can and aim to grab your right hand. Hold.

Step 7

Undo the pose slowly and repeat it with the arms and legs in the reverse position.

Chakra: Svadisthana

Benefits:

- Reduced resistance to life.
- Increased sexuality and sensuality
- Reduced tension headaches
- Improved pelvic movement
- Reduced menstrual pain and fluctuations

Downward Facing Dog- Adho Mukha Svasana

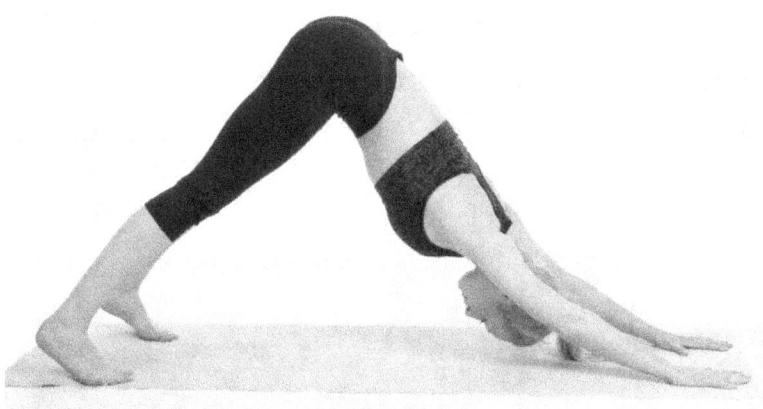

Description:

Starting Position

Start on your hands and knees with your wrists under your shoulders and your knees under your hips. Spread your fingers wide and tuck your toes under. Inhale.

Step 1

Exhale and push your hips up to the ceiling. Straighten your legs as much as possible. If your heels are off the floor, try stepping forward to give yourself a sturdier base. Aim to keep your head between your arms and look back between your legs. Keep your tailbone pushed towards the ceiling and hold.

Step 2

Release by bending the knees and dropping back onto your hands and knees into Child's pose. Rest and repeat three times.

If this position is too strong you may find it easier to drop your elbows and forearms to the floor. Alternatively, hold the back of a chair and step backwards until your torso is parallel to the floor and your feet are hip width apart.

Chakra: Sahasrara

Benefits:

- Increased bone density and stronger hands and wrists
- Increased flexibility and strength in the lower legs
- Reduced back pain and tension through elongating the cervical spine
- Increased blood circulation and vitality
- Improved respiration

Reduced anxiety.

Chapter 5

Yoga for inner peace

As we discussed in the previous chapter, stress can have a huge effect on our state of mind. It can generate a wide range of negative emotions such as anger, frustration, depression and anxiety. When we hold onto these emotions our internal balance can become quite unstable and we lose control. Alternatively they may develop and fester to the point where we find it hard to experience positive emotions. We just feel bad all the time and we struggle to connect with the world around us.

This kind of internal stress can originate from many sources including communication breakdowns with family, friends and coworkers, anxiety about financial situations, feelings of inadequacy and low self-esteem.

Physical issues occur when these emotions have no outlet and they build up inside us. They are just as damaging as toxins to our body and can literally make us sick.

Yoga provides an outlet for this pent up negative energy and helps us to rebuild our internal balance. As we move though the postures and rest between them we have time for the mind to bring all our thoughts and feelings to the surface where we can observe the effect they have on our bodies.

As a newcomer to yoga, you might find it very hard to relax at first as your body holds on tightly to all the strong emotions within you. You may find that your thoughts keep returning to the source of your stress even when your body is in a relaxed position. Slowing down your breathing may also be difficult. This is a normal experience so don't worry about it or try to fight it.

Instead, as you become aware of your negative thought, try and simply observe and acknowledge that it is there but try not to get drawn into it. Imagine you are looking at it impassively from arm's length. Then once you have accepted that it is there, let it float away and try and bring your thoughts back to your breathing and your internal energy flow. This will take practice but it is well worth persisting as you will soon be able to gain more control of your emotions and remain calm for longer periods.

Eventually you will find that you are able to handle everyday situations more easily and you can retain clarity and focus. Continued practice of yoga in any form helps to develop a general sense of peace and well-being. You will find that your positive emotions are back in the forefront and although the negative aspects of life are still there, you will be in a much better state of mind to deal with them.

These postures help to induce a sense of calm and well-being.

Child's Pose - Balasana

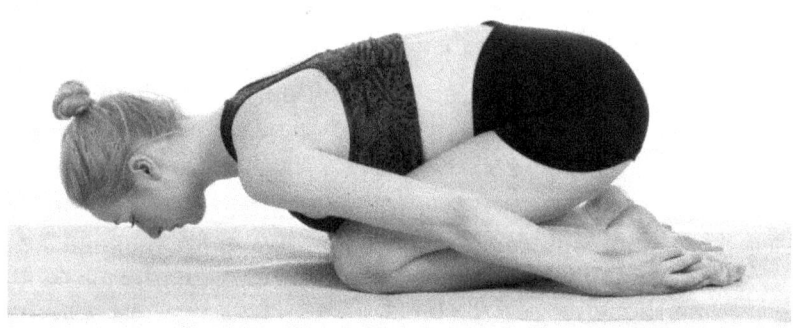

Description:

This pose can be used as a resting pose after back bending-postures or anytime you need to calm your body down and relax. It is great for winding down after a busy day.

Starting Position

Start on your hands and knees with your wrists under your shoulders and your knees slightly wider than your hips. Point the toes and keep the tops of your feet against the floor. Inhale.

Step 1

Exhale and gently raise your head and torso upright as you sit back onto your heels with your hands on your thighs.

Step 2

Inhale and raise both hands to the ceiling with the palms facing forward.

Step 3

Exhale and slowly bend forward from the hips. Lower your hands to the floor in front of you with the palms down and the arms extended forward.

Allow the chest to rest on top of the thighs. Aim to have the forehead touching the floor and the buttocks resting on the heels. If needed, create two fists, place them one above the other and rest your forehead on them for support.

Alternatively you can bring the arms down beside the body with the palms up and the fingers pointing towards the toes. Once you are comfortable, gradually let all the tension in your body drain away as though you were melting. Close your eyes and breathe into this position.

Step 4

When you are ready, slowly push yourself upright into a kneeling position then bring your legs around to the front and stretch them out. Give them a little shake to loosen any tightness.

Chakra: Anahata

Benefits:

- More flexibility in the hips, ankles, thighs and lower back
- Greater awareness of the breath and the flow of energy through the body

- Increased sense of calm which can continue for some time
- Increased balance between the heart and the mind
- Reduced symptoms of heart and lung conditions

Happy Baby Pose - Ananda Balasana

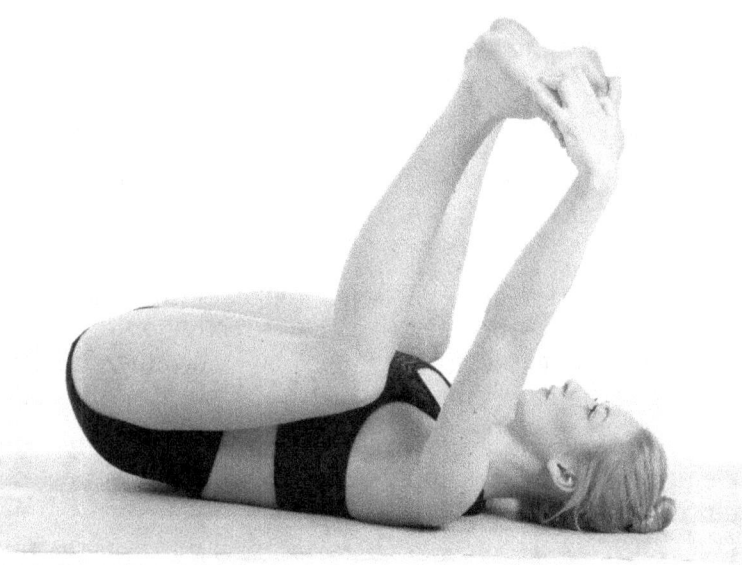

Description:

This pose is helpful for those who are unwell or have physical limitations as it can also be done while lying in bed.

Starting Position

Begin by lying on your back then draw your knees up to the chest while you exhale.

Step 1

Grip either the outsides of your feet or your big toes depending on your level of comfort and flexibility. Inhale and raise the soles of your feet towards the ceiling keeping your ankles in line above your knees. Push your knees towards your armpits.

Step 2

Gently flex your heels upwards and push against your hands while your hands offer firm resistance. Hold.

Step 3

Release by lowering your feet to the floor then stretch out on your back. Repeat three times then rest in Corpse pose.

Chakra: Svadisthana

Benefits:

- Improved hip strength and flexibility
- Reduced pain and tension in the thighs, pelvis and lower back
- Increased sense of calm and positive energy
- Reduced fatigue
- Increased acceptance and relaxed resistance to life
- Increased sensuality and sexuality

Head to Knee Forward Bend – Janu Sirsasana

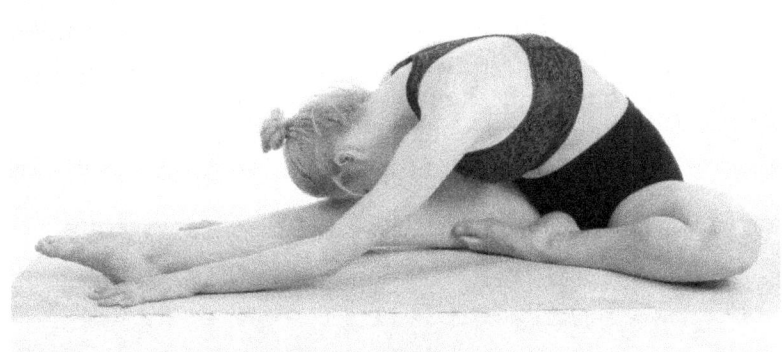

Description:

Starting Position

Sit on the floor with your legs out in front of you.

Step 1

Bend the right knee and place the sole of that foot flat against the inside of the left thigh. Aim to keep the right knee on the floor.

Step 2

Turn your head and torso towards the left so that your naval is in line with your extended left leg.

Step 3

Inhale and stretch both arms out to the sides then swing them up towards the ceiling.

Step 4

Exhale and lean forward and down over the left leg, leading with the chin. Sweep your hands down to grab your lower leg or foot as far down as you can reach.

Step 5

Inhale again and lift the head and chest while maintaining your grip. Then as you exhale, drop the head, bend the elbows and reach forward while pushing your tailbone down.

Aim to place your palms on the floor and your head on your knee. Keep your head down and gradually inch further forward on each exhalation. Hold.

Step 6

When you are ready, slowly raise your head and sternum and drag your hands along the leg until you are upright. Use your hands to support the right knee and place your right foot flat on the floor. Straighten the legs and wiggle them around to loosen any tension. Take several full breaths and repeat the posture on the opposite side.

Chakra: Muladhara and Svadisthana

Benefits:

- Increased sense of calm and well-being
- Reduced symptoms of mild depression, insomnia, anxiety, headaches and sinusitis
- Improved digestion and waste elimination
- Improved hormonal balance
- Reduced high blood pressure
- Greater strength and flexibility through the whole body

Tree Pose – Vrksasana

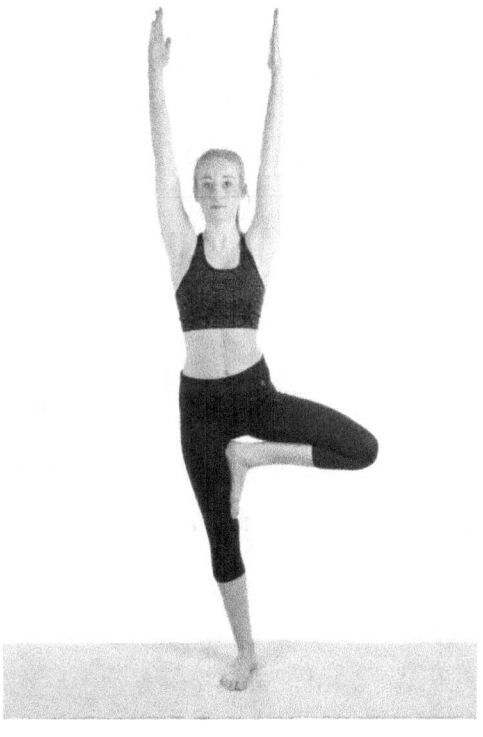

Description:

Starting Position

Start in Mountain pose then transfer your weight over the left foot.

Step 1

Bend your right knee, reach down with your right hand and grab the right ankle. Bring it up and place the sole of that foot against the inner left thigh or calf. Keep the left arm out as a counterbalance. To help maintain your balance, focus on a fixed point several feet in front of you at eye level.

Step 2

Once you are steady place your hands in front of your chest in Prayer pose and push the palms together. You may choose to stay in this position.

Step 3

Alternatively, reach your arms out to the sides for balance then inhale and lift them above your head. Stretch your fingers up to the ceiling with the palms forward. Hold.

Step 4

When you are ready, drop your leg and hands down so you are back in Mountain pose. Rest and then repeat the posture on your opposite leg.

Chakra: Muladhara

Benefits:

- Increased sense of security and being grounded
- Increased physical, mental and emotional balance
- Improved focus and concentration
- Reduced pressure from sciatica
- Firmer thighs, calves and abdominal muscles

Corpse Pose – Savasana

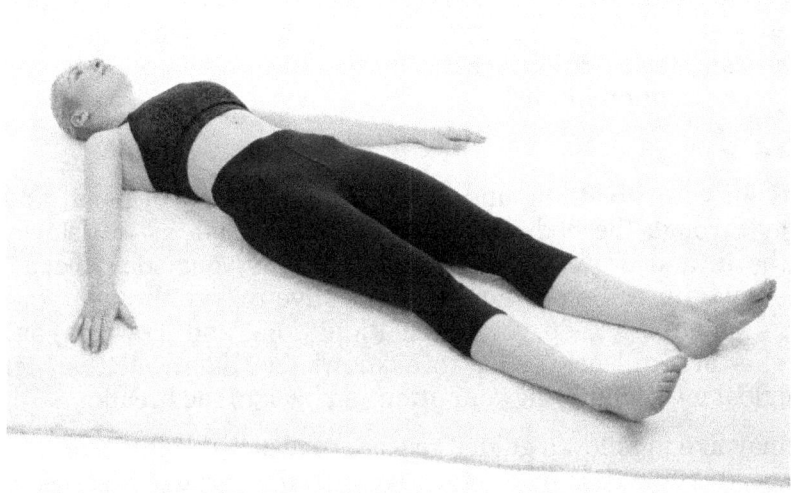

Description:

This posture can be used as a rest in between other floor based postures, during meditation or at the end of a full yoga session

Starting Position

Begin in a seated position with your legs straight out in front and slightly apart. Place your hands on the floor just behind the hips

Step 1

Bend your elbows and slowly lower your torso and head to the floor. Stretch your arms out to either side slightly away from body. Rest your palms up with the fingers relaxed and slightly curled. Turn the wrists outwards a little and let your feet flop out to the sides.

Step 2

Focus on the alignment of your spine, hips and shoulders. Imagine a straight line running from the crown of your head though the body and ending at a point centered between the feet. Drop your shoulders back and down, elongate the neck and crown, tilt your pelvis up towards the navel and pull the tailbone towards the feet.

Step 3

Close your eyes and open the mouth slightly. Let your tongue rest loosely behind the lower front teeth, relax the facial and jaw muscles and feel your whole scalp loosen. Rest in this position and turn your attention inwards.

Step 4

Focus on your breathing and be aware of the flow of blood and energy through the body. Expand your diaphragm as you slowly breathe in and draw positive energy towards your solar plexus. Then as you breathe out expel any negative energy through your fingers and toes. Keep your exhalations long and slow. If your thoughts are still active, try to acknowledge them but then let them float away and bring your attention back to the breath.

You may like to follow a guided relaxation exercise at this point. In a class situation your instructor may talk you through a series of mental exercises that focus on relaxing the body in sequence from your head to your toes. At home you can play a pre-recorded audio file of a guided relaxation, listen to some soothing music or simply enjoy the silence.

Step 5

To come out of the pose, gradually wiggle your fingers and toes followed by your larger joints then when you are ready, open your eyes and blink a few times.

Raise your right arm above your head, roll onto your right side and place your left hand on the floor in front of you. Push your left hand into the floor, draw your right elbow under your torso then lift and turn into a comfortable sitting position. Allow your focus to return to the present and your heart rate to steady before attempting to stand.

Chakra: All chakras

Benefits:

- Reduced stress, anxiety and depression

- Increased vitality and overall sense of well-being
- Reduced intensity and frequency of headaches, fatigue and insomnia
- Improved focus and concentration
- Improved sense of balance and of feeling grounded

Chapter 6

A 12 step daily routine you can do in minutes.

Salute to the Sun – Surya Namaskar

This series of 12 postures is one of the most popular and versatile posture sequences practiced in yoga today. It is also called "Good Morning" or "Sun Salutation". The postures can be performed by a beginner but are beneficial for even the most advanced of yogis. There are a number of variations to each posture but the basic ones have been included here.

If you don't have enough time to go to the gym or for a run, you can still do 3 rounds of this routine in less than 10 minutes each morning at home.

The "Salute to the Sun" sequence is a complete routine of physical fitness and relaxation in itself. It works every muscle, joint and major organ in the body and also stimulates the breathing and circulation. Every chakra is activated providing emotional balance and a sense of serenity.

- Steps 1 and 12 promote focus and awareness
- Steps 2 and 11 expand the chest and fill the body with energy
- Steps 3 and 10 massage the internal organs and improve digestion
- Steps 4 and 9 strengthen the ankles, knees and hips
- Steps 5 and 8 stretch and tone the entire body from top to toe
- Steps 6 and 7 expand the chest, tone the body, relieve fatigue and stimulate the nervous system, kidneys and adrenal glands.

Note that in the "Low Lunge" (Steps 4 and 9), the right leg goes back and the left leg comes forward in Step 4. However in Step 9 the left leg goes back and the right leg comes forward. This is to ensure both sides are stretched evenly.

To begin with you may find it difficult to get into these postures and hold them. Don't worry; as long as you aim to get a bit better each time and don't force any position you will still reap the benefits of yoga.

As you learn the routine, say the step numbers to yourself. Aim for a continuous, fluid motion and try not to pause in between each posture.

Performing this sequence as a habit each morning will give you a huge boost of energy to sustain you though the day. Over time you will find you have greater agility and endurance physically and a calmer, more balanced outlook on life.

Step 1

Mountain Pose and Prayer Pose – Tadasana and Pranamasana

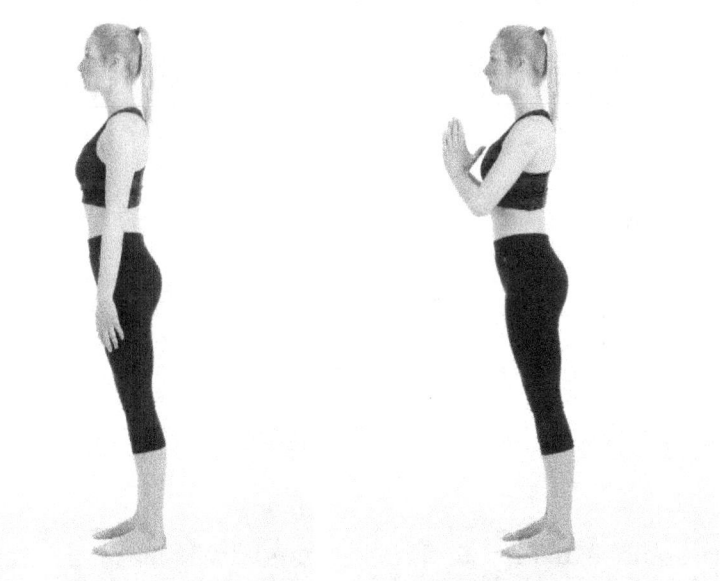

This step merges two poses into one fluid movement.

Begin by standing with the feet slightly apart, the hands relaxed by the sides, the head facing forward and the spine in full alignment. Check your weight is distributed evenly and the soles of your feet are spread flat to the floor. This is known as Mountain Pose and it is also used as a neutral position when moving between many other poses.

Inhale and lift your arms out to the sides then above your head in one continuous movement. Finish with the palms against each other.

Exhale and bring the hands down in front of your chest with your palms pushing against each other and your elbows out to the side. Briefly drop your head to your chest then look forward again. This hand position is known as Prayer Pose.

Step 2

Upward Salute – Urdhva Hastasana

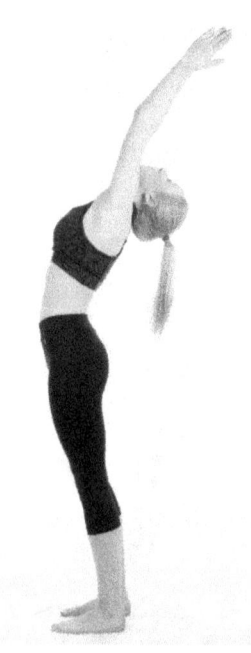

Inhale and extend your arms up and back as far as you can, keeping the biceps close to the ears. Use the fingers to extend the stretch rather than the lower back. Expand your chest and engage your whole body in the stretch.

Step 3

Standing Forward Bend - Uttanasana

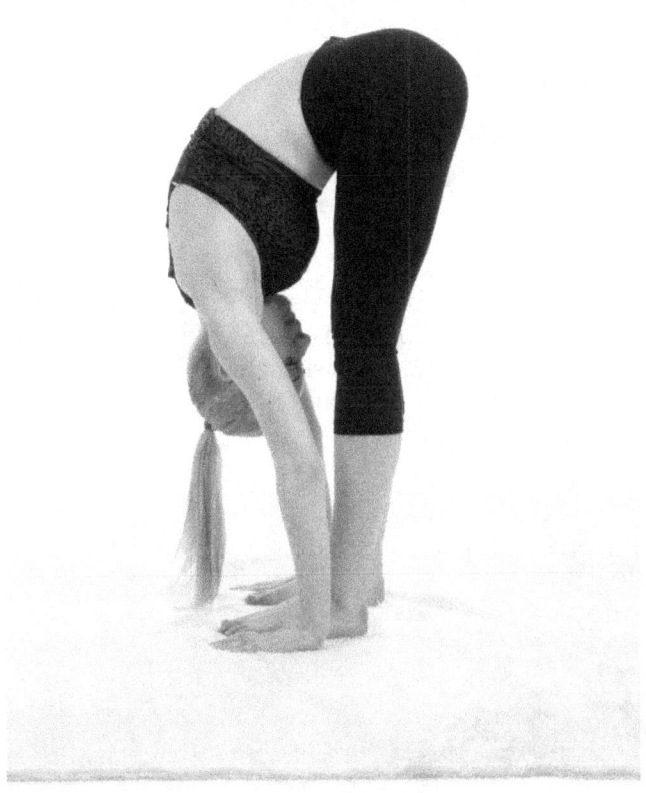

Exhale and gently drop forward keeping your arms extended and the spine straight. Bend from the waist and aim to bring your nose to your knees and the hands flat to the floor alongside the feet.

You can bend the knees slightly to get the hands to the floor and then straighten the legs again. Try not to move your hands from this position throughout the next few poses.

Step 4

Low Lunge - Ashwa Sanchalanasana

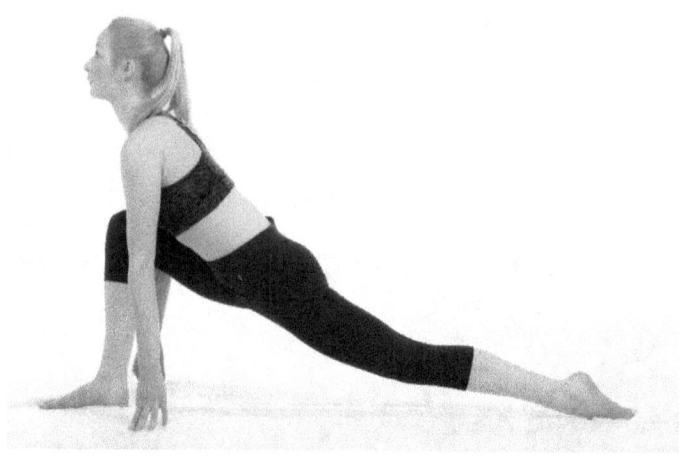

Inhale and extend your right leg backwards as far as possible with the top of the foot against the floor. Drop the right knee to the floor and lift your head up by leading with the chin. Check that your left foot is centered between your hands.

Step 5

Plank - Chaturanga

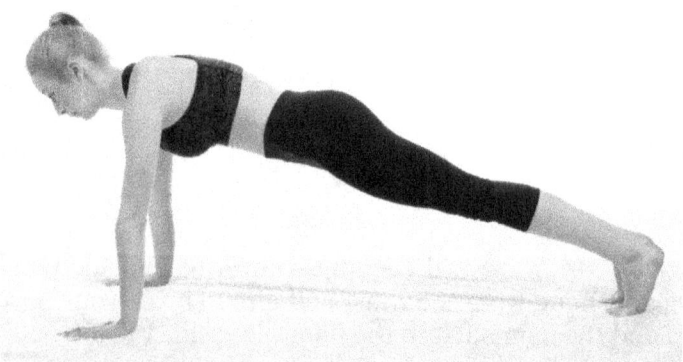

This pose is also known as the "Four-Limbed Staff".

Inhale and extend the left leg back alongside the right. Lower your head so that your crown, back and legs are in a straight line. Take your weight on your toes and palms and keep your elbows straight.

Step 6

Salute with Eight Limbs Pose - Ashtanga Namaskara

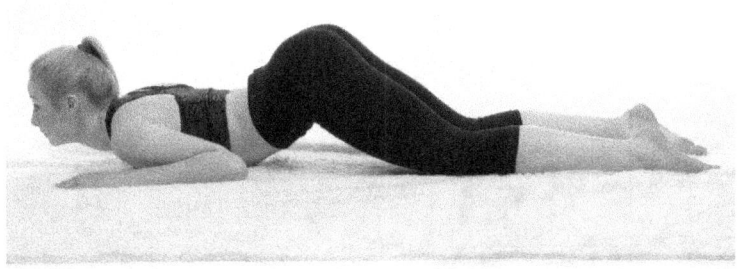

This pose is sometimes known as "Knees, Chest and Chin" or "Caterpillar". The "Eight Limbs" in the pose name are the two hands, two feet, two knees, chest and chin.

In one continuous exhalation, gently lower your knees to the floor, push your buttocks back over your heels and keep your arms extended forward in a brief Child's pose.

In the same movement come forward onto your knees, sweep the chest forward to the floor between the hands, raise the buttocks towards the ceiling and put your chin on the floor.

Step 7

Cobra – Bhujangasana

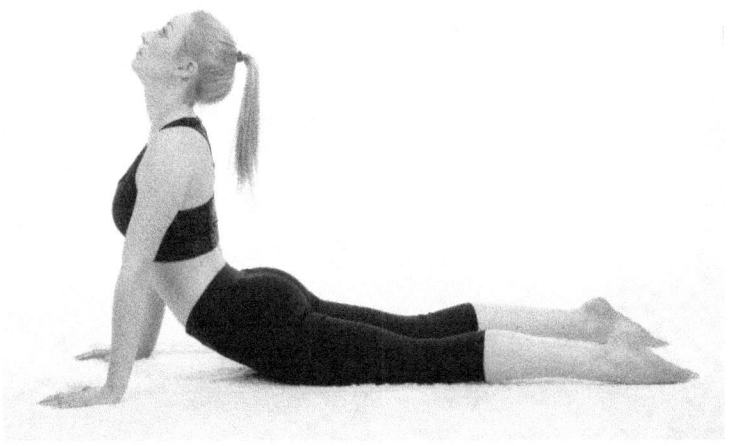

Inhale and slide the chest forward, up and back then let your head drop back slightly. Keep your shoulders back and down and aim to straighten the arms.

Step 8

Downward Facing Dog – Adho Mukha Svanasana

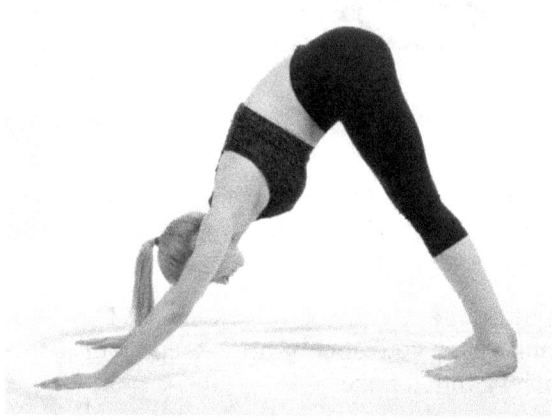

Tuck your toes under and as you exhale push the buttocks up towards the ceiling and stretch into an inverted 'V' posture. Aim to keep your heels on the floor. Keep your ears next to your upper arms and look back towards your shins.

Step 9

Low Lunge - Ashwa Sanchalanasana

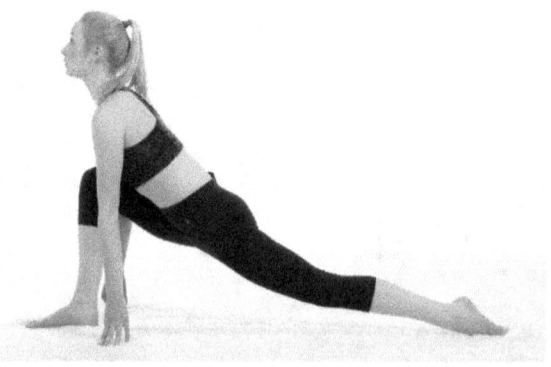

This is the same pose as Step 4. However this time you are stretching the other side of the body.

From the previous position, inhale and step the right leg forward with the right foot between the hands and the right knee bent near the chest. Drop the left knee to the floor and lift your head up by leading with the chin.

Step 10

Standing Forward Bend – Uttanasana

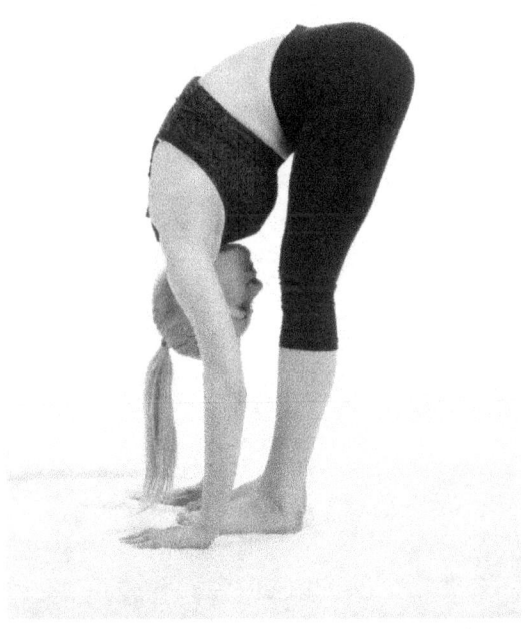

This is the same pose as Step 3.

Exhale and step the left foot forward keeping your arms extended and the spine straight. Bend from the waist and aim to bring your nose to your knees and the hands flat to the floor alongside the feet. You can bend the knees slightly to get the hands to the floor and then straighten the knees again.

Step 11

Upward Salute – Urdhva Hastasana

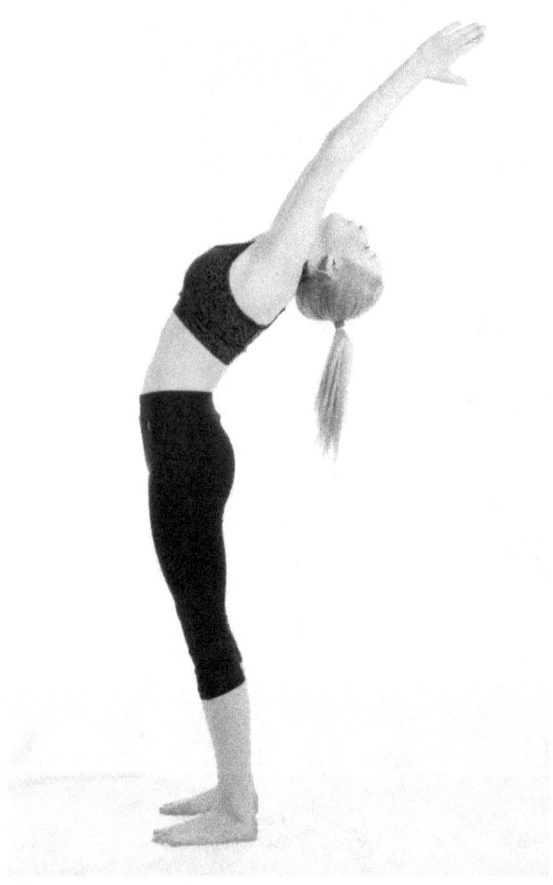

This is the same pose as Step 2.

Inhale and extend your arms up and back as far as you can, keeping the biceps close to the ears. Use the fingers to extend the stretch rather than the lower back. Expand your chest and engage your whole body in the stretch.

Step 12

Mountain Pose and Prayer Pose – Tadasana and Pranamasana

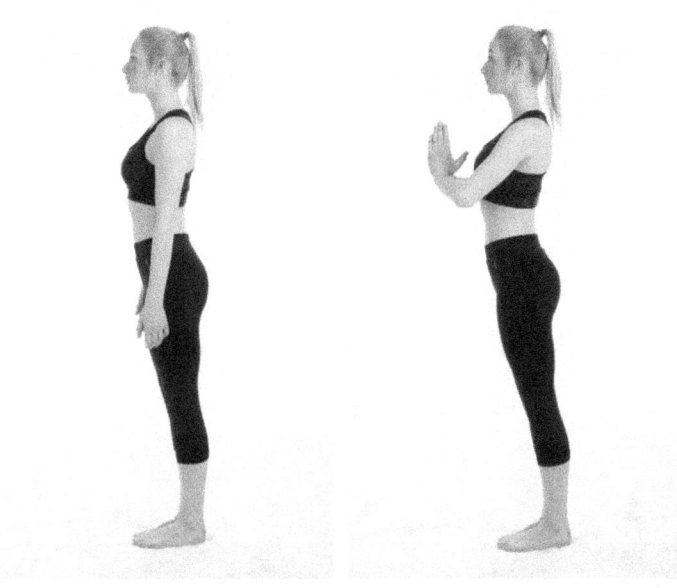

Exhale and as your torso comes forward, stretch your arms out to the sides then complete the arc by swinging the arms down to the sides with the palms to the thighs.

Inhale and sweep the palms up over the abdomen until the palms meet in Prayer pose. At the same time, curl the spine and neck back slightly. On the exhalation, briefly drop your head to your chest then look forward again. Inhale and smile as you release the position then exhale and relax the body.

Chapter 7

10 Classic Yoga Postures

These can be done in isolation or in sequence with a pause in between.

1. *Yoga Mudra*

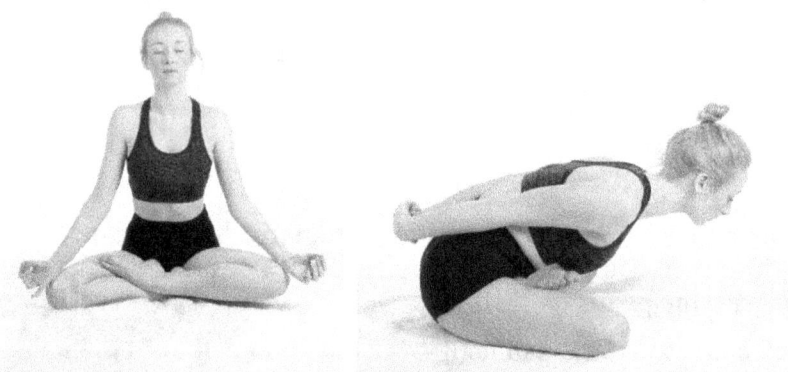

Description:

The term 'mudra' means 'seal' and in yoga terms it signifies a ring or joining. There are many forms of mudras in yoga including Hasta (hand), Mana (mind) and Kaya (body). In each case they represent a union of some kind that facilitates the flow of energy through the body. They are often combined with various postures and also with focused thoughts or affirmations.

Mudras are generally performed three times. The first is for the self, the second is for others and the third is for the universe. This posture uses the Gyan hand mudra which is for knowledge, concentration or memory. The affirmation is based on acceptance.

Starting Position

Sit in a comfortable cross-legged position.

Step 1

Place the hands over the knees with the palms up. Join the tips of the index fingers and the thumbs to create an "O" shape (Gyan Mudra) and let the other fingers uncurl loosely.

Step 2

While maintaining this hand mudra, drop the hands to the floor on either side of the knees and sweep the fingers back along the floor until they meet at the base of the spine.

Step 3

Grasp the wrists together and push them up the back as far as you can.

Step 4

Inhale and then on the exhalation lean forward with the chin and chest and try to avoid hunching the spine. Bring the chest to rest on the thighs and lastly drop the head down. Hold.

Step 5

To release the position, use your hips to swing the torso upright. Drop the back of the hands to the floor, inhale and sweep them along the floor to the knees back into the Gyan hand mudra.

At the same time lift the sternum and drop the head back slightly. Exhale and face forward with your hands cupped over the knees.

Step 6

Repeat this posture three times. During the first time, focus your thoughts on accepting all aspects of yourself. During the second time, focus on accepting others and during the third focus on accepting the universe and acknowledging your place in it.

Chakra: All chakras

Benefits:

- Increased acceptance of the self and others

- Increased focus and mental clarity
- Greater flexibility in the spine and hips
- More balanced emotions

2. Seated Spine Twist – Ardha Matsyendrasana

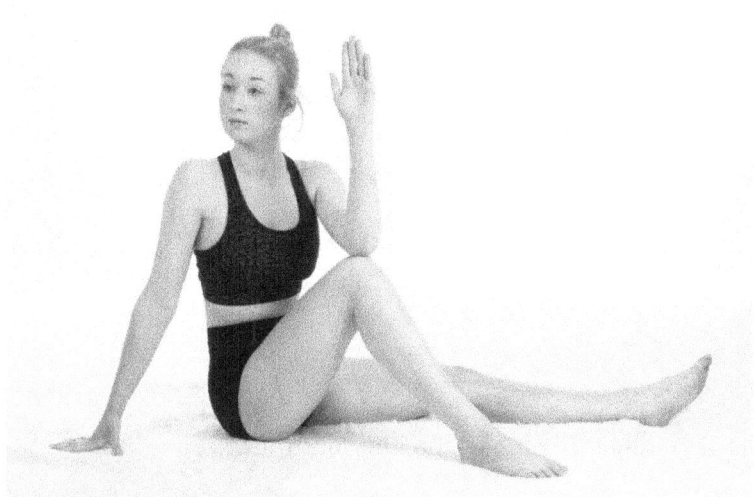

Description:

Starting Position

Sit upright with both legs straight out in front of you.

Step 1

Bend the left knee and slide the foot up alongside the right knee.

Step 2

Inhale and swing the right arm to the ceiling. As you exhale bring it down in an arc to cup the left knee with the right hand. Alternatively, hook the right elbow over the left knee.

Step 3

Inhale and raise the left arm to the ceiling then exhale and swing it back tight behind the left hip. Place the palm on the floor with fingers pointing away from the body.

Step 4

Turn the head to the left then follow with your torso to create a lateral twist. Push with your hands to extend the twist and keep your torso raised out of the hips. Hold.

Step 5

To release the pose, turn the head to the front then swing your right arm in an arc above your head and place it beside the right hip.

Then swing your left arm back behind you, raise it in an arc above your head then drop it forward and down to rest beside the left hip. Face forward, straighten your legs and wiggle them a little. Repeat on your opposite side.

Chakra: Muladhara, Svadisthana and Manipura

Benefits:

- Increased circulation to all spinal nerves, veins and tissues
- Improved spinal strength and flexibility
- Calmer nervous system
- Reduced lower back pain

3. Bridge Pose – Setu Bandha Sarvangasana

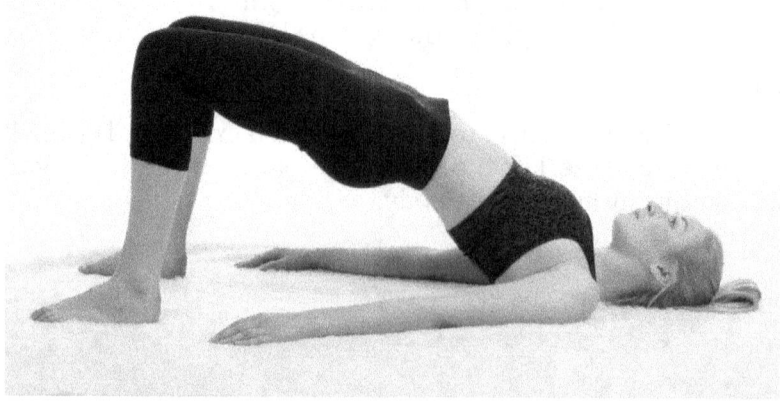

Description:

Starting Position

Begin by lying on your back with your hands by your sides.

Step 1

Inhale and bend your knees while drawing your feet up towards the hips as closely as possible. Keep your arms on the floor or grab your ankles if you can reach them.

Step 2

As you exhale, raise your hips up off the floor as high as you can while arching the back. To support your back you can either clasp your hands together and push the arms against the floor or you can bend your elbows and place your hands under your hips.

Step 3

Lift your navel up towards the ceiling and elongate the spine through the backbend. It may help to imagine that someone has a string tied to your navel and is pulling it straight up. Feel the body fall naturally back into an arch. Hold.

Step 4

To come down, gently roll the spine down onto the floor using your arms for balance and support. Repeat three times.

Step 5

Draw the knees up to the chest and hug them to release any tension on the back. You may want to roll around a little in this position. Then bring your feet back to the floor, stretch out on your back and relax in Corpse pose.

Chakra: Svadisthana and Manipura

Benefits:

- Stronger and firmer leg, abdominal, chest and back muscles
- Stronger bones and reduced risk of osteoporosis

- Calmer disposition and reduced stress and anxiety

- Reduced menstrual and menopausal symptoms

- Reduced back pain, headaches and tired legs

- Improved digestion and energy through stimulation of the abdomen, chest and thyroid

- Improved asthma, blood pressure and sinusitis

4. Seated Forward Bend – Pashimotanasana

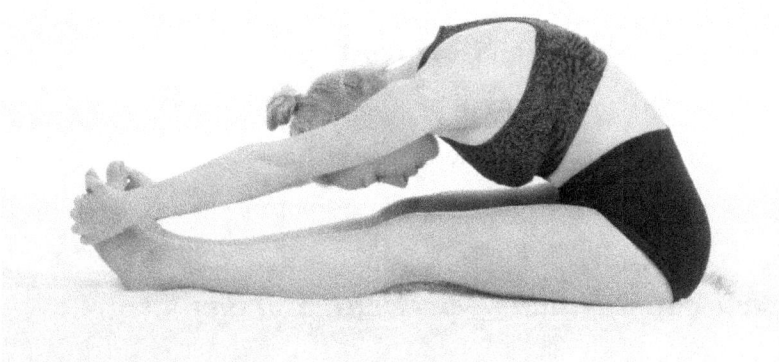

Description:

Starting Position

Begin by sitting with both legs out in front, feet together and your hands beside your hips.

Step 1

Inhale and rotate your arms back in an arc behind the body, up towards the ceiling and then forward to the knees. Use this momentum to slide your hands forward along your shins and to bend forward from the hips.

Step 2

Exhale and reach your hands forward to clasp the outsides of the feet allowing the head to drop forward. If you can't reach that far, grip the ankles or sides of the legs instead. Breathe into the upper chest and with each exhalation, aim to lower yourself further. Hold.

Step 3

To release the posture, inhale and slide your hands back up along the legs to the thighs. Use your abdominal muscles to slowly uncurl the body leaving your head until last. Repeat three times then lie on your back and relax in Corpse pose.

Chakra: Muladhara and Svadisthana

Benefits:
- Improved kidney and liver function
- Improved symptoms of menopause and menstruation
- Reduced anxiety and depression
- Stronger muscles in the back, groin and legs

5. Upward Abdominal Lock - Uddiyana Bandha

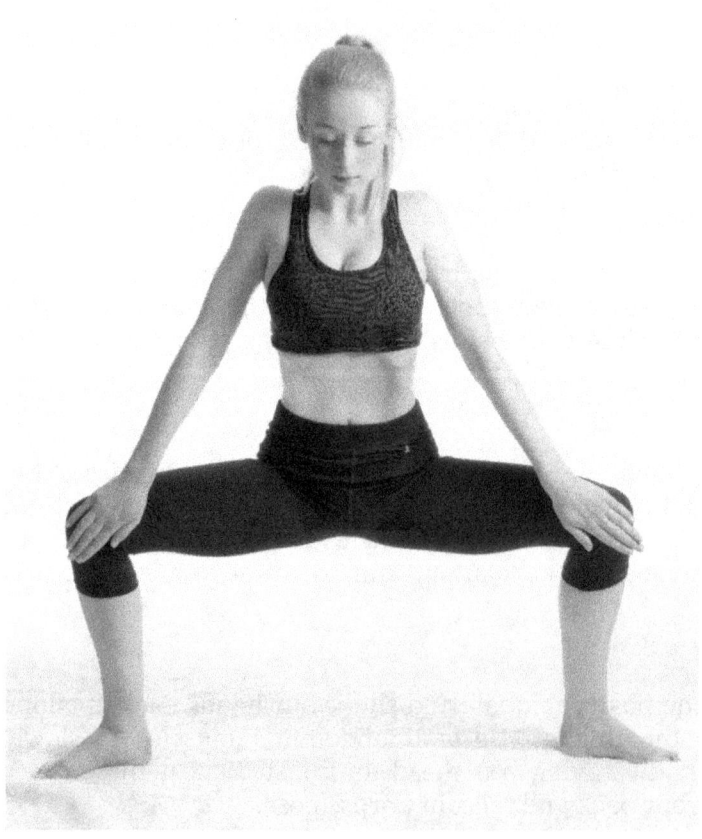

Description:

Starting Position

Stand up straight in Mountain pose.

Step 1

Part the legs wide and point the toes outwards. Press the tailbone down into a wide squat and place the hands on the thighs.

Step 2

Breathe in deeply through the nose then exhale quickly through the mouth while drawing the abdomen back, up and under creating a lock in the groin.

Tuck the chin to the chest and create another lock in the throat. Hold without breath for as long as you can.

Step 3

When you need to release, inhale and drop into a loose forward bend. Let the body hang until the breath returns to normal. Repeat three times.

Chakra: Muladhara and Visuddha

Benefits:

- Improved symptoms of constipation and indigestion
- Stronger abdominal muscles and diaphragm
- Stimulated blood circulation in the abdomen
- Reduced thyroid disturbances
- Improved elimination of toxins

6. Locust – Shalabasana

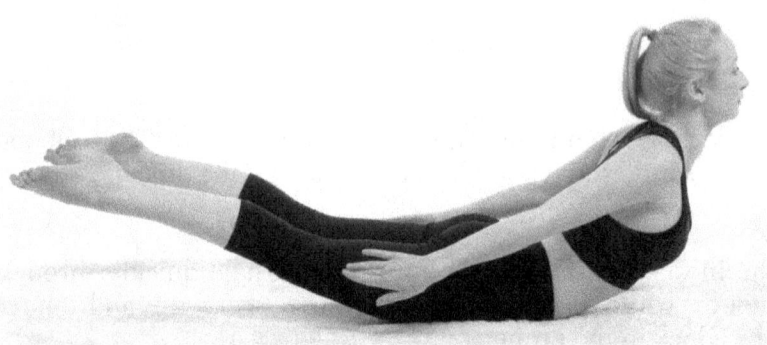

Description:

Starting Position

Begin by lying on your stomach with your forehead resting on the floor and your hands by your sides, palms facing up.

Step 1

Inhale and push your heels towards each other.

Step 2

Exhale and raise your legs, thighs, chest and head off the floor in a backwards arc. Keep your head facing forward and lift the crown of the head up.

Step 3

Lift your arms so they are parallel to the floor and stretch your fingers back, palms up. Point your toes and keep your legs straight.

Extend the stretch along the back of the body from the toes to the crown and balance your weight on your belly. Hold.

Step 4

Release by lowering your legs, arms and head to the floor. Turn your head to one side with your ear to the floor while your breathing slows down. Repeat three times.

Chakra: All chakras

Benefits:
- Reduced stress and body tension
- Reduced symptoms of indigestion and flatulence
- Improved posture
- Improved drive and determination
- Firmer muscles in the legs, buttocks, spine and arms

7. Cobra – Bhujangasana

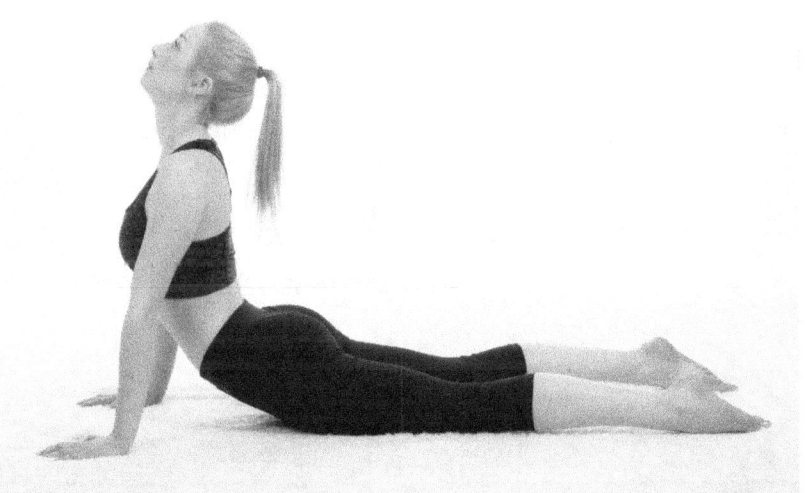

Description:

Starting Position

Lie face down with your forehead on the floor and your arms by your sides.

Step 1

Place your palms on the floor under your shoulders, tuck the elbows inwards and push your heels towards each other.

Step 2

Inhale and slowly raise your head and chest leaving your elbows and forearms on the floor. Lift up through the sternum while you arch your lower back. Allow the head to drop back. Keep your thighs on the floor and only lift as high as you feel comfortable.

Alternatively, place your hands flat on the floor alongside the chest with the elbows up towards the ceiling before you lift and straighten the arms out. Hold.

Step 3

Use your arms to gently lower yourself back to the floor then rest your arms by your sides. Turn your head to one side with your ear to the floor while your breathing slows down. Repeat three times.

Chakra: Muladhara, Svadisthana and Manipura

Benefits:

- Reduced symptoms of sciatica and asthma
- Tighter abdominal muscles
- Increased energy and sense of well-being
- Improved digestion and metabolism
- Reduced resistance to change

8. Supported Shoulder Stand – Salamba Sarvangasana

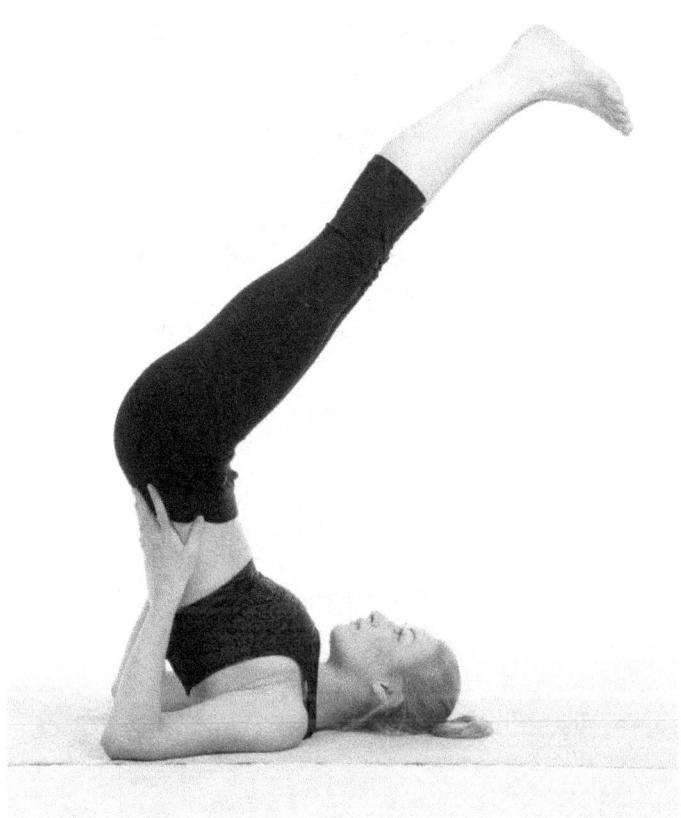

Description:

Starting Position

Sit upright with your legs out in front and your knees slightly bent. Place your fists on the floor beside your hips.

Step 1

Breathe in and lean forward a little then quickly roll the whole body back along the spine. Use your fists to push against the floor and also use your abdominal muscles to lift the buttocks up in the air above the chest. Exhale as you straighten your legs and aim to touch your toes to the floor above your head.

Step 2

Bring your hands up to support your upper back as close to the neck as you can and draw your elbows in tight for support. This position is known and the Plough Pose and you can remain there instead of going into a full shoulder stand if you want to.

Step 3

From Plough pose, bend your knees and draw them up so they rest on your forehead with your feet in the air.

Step 4

Inhale and straighten your legs towards the ceiling with your toes flexed and your heels pushing upwards. Aim to create a straight line from your heels through your torso to your upper back. Lift your upper back away from the floor as high as you can and use your arms for support. Hold.

Step 5

To come out of the posture exhale, drop your knees back to your forehead and your arms to the floor. Very gently roll your spine down, taking care not to lift your head off the floor, until you are lying on your back. Always follow this pose immediately with Fish pose.

Chakra: Anahata, Visuddha and Ajna

Benefits:

- Improved function of the thyroid and prostate glands
- Strengthened neck and shoulders
- More toned legs and buttocks
- Reduced symptoms of anxiety, depression, fatigue and insomnia
- Stimulated imagination, intuition and creativity
- Improved ability to communicate clearly

9. Fish – Matsyasana

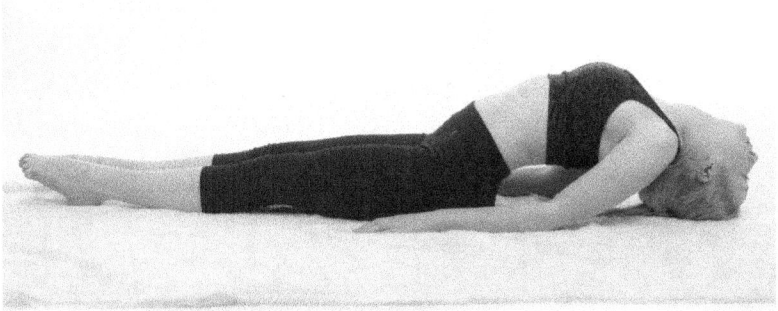

Description:

The Fish is a counter pose to the shoulder stand and the two are normally performed together.

Starting Position

Lie flat on the back with the hands under the buttocks and the palms down.

Step 1

Spread the thumbs away from the index fingers and position them in a 'V' shape around your sitting bones. Tuck your elbows in tight under the chest.

Step 2

Inhale and slowly raise your diaphragm and solar plexus towards the ceiling, drawing your shoulder blades towards each other and letting the neck and head follow.

Depending on how high you lift, either your crown or the back of your head will be on the floor but do not take any weight on your head. Instead, distribute your weight evenly along your forearms and point your toes away as a counterbalance. Hold.

Step 3

To release the position, exhale, bring your shoulders down and gently lower your back to the floor.

Step 4

Place your feet flat on the floor and slide them away to straighten the legs. Relax in Corpse pose until your breathing returns to normal.

Chakra: Anahata, Visuddha and Ajna

Benefits:

- Improved symptoms of respiratory disorders
- Reduced back and menstrual pain
- Improved digestion
- Stronger muscles along the back and neck
- Improved creativity and intuition
- Increased perception and general awareness

10. Half Head Stand – Ardha Sirsasana

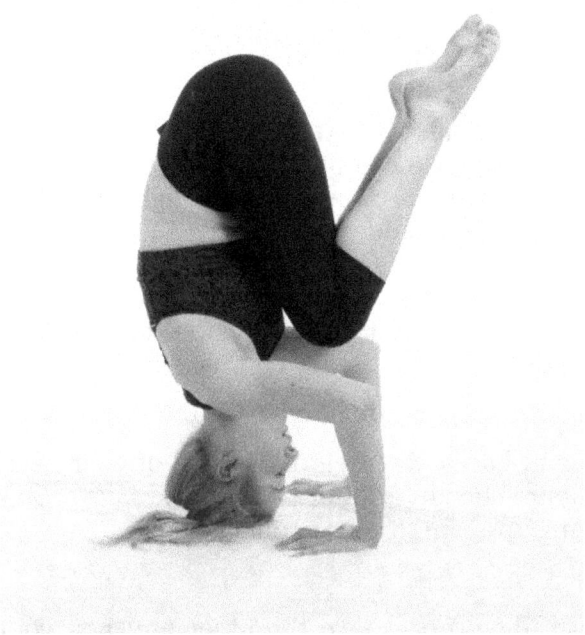

Description:

There are a number of variations of this posture. This basic variation is sometimes called the "Teddy Bear".

Starting Position

Start on your hands and knees with your wrists under your shoulders, your knees under your hips and your toes tucked under. Your palms should be spread flat and facing forward.

Step 1

Gently lean forward and place the crown of your head on the floor to form a tripod base with your hands. You may need to shift around a little to find a balance point. Your forearms should now be at right angles to the floor.

Step 2

Inhale and straighten your knees so your tailbone is raised towards the ceiling.

Step 3

Walk your toes forward until your knees touch your elbows.

Step 4

Slowly place the left knee up onto the left elbow, lifting the foot off the floor. Then place the right knee onto the right elbow. Touch your toes together for stability. Keep your weight centered between your crown and palms. Hold.

Step 5

To come down, extend one leg and place that foot on the floor followed by the opposite leg.

Step 6

Drop to your hands and knees. Sit back on the top of your heels leaving your arms outstretched in front of you in Child's pose. Stay there briefly then swing up again to your hands and knees.

Step 7

Create two fists, place them one above the other and rest your forehead on them for support. Lower your buttocks onto your heels with the tops of your feet to the floor. Remain in this position until your breath returns to normal.

Step 8

Sit up on your heels and place your hands on your thighs. Drop your head to your chest and gently roll it from side to side.

Lift your head back to a neutral position and then slowly look over your left shoulder and then your right shoulder.

Return to the neutral position and very carefully drop your head back with your mouth open and your chin towards the ceiling.

If you can, very slowly move your head from side to side to relieve any tension in the neck. Return to the center and carefully raise your head back to neutral and face forward.

Shrug your shoulders a few times and then lie down on your back and relax in Corpse pose.

Chakra: Ajna and Sahasrara

Benefits:

- Improved balance
- Greater control of thoughts and actions
- Improved cognitive ability
- Increased blood supply to the brain
- Improved imagination and intuition
- Stronger muscles in shoulders and neck

Always end a yoga session with a form of relaxation to allow the body to warm down. You may want to cover yourself with a blanket and use a small pillow for comfort. You can practice some deep breathing exercises or follow a spoken guided relaxation. Your instructor may do this in a class situation or you can listen to one of the countless audio files available online.

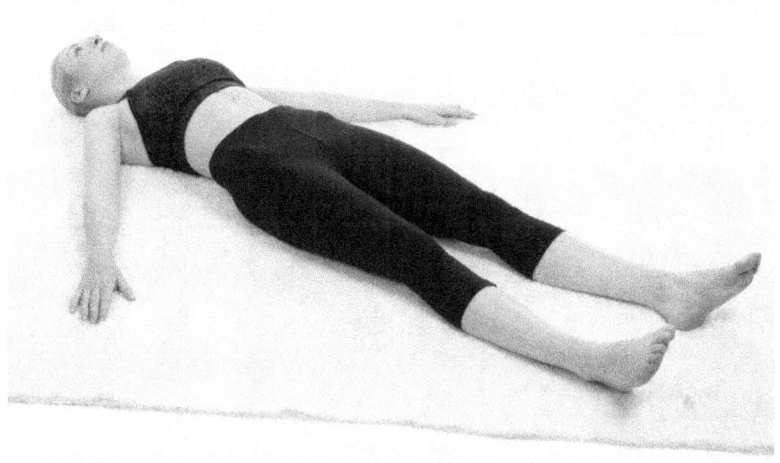

See Chapter 5 for the description and benefits of Corpse pose.

Conclusion

I hope this book was able to help you understand the benefits of yoga and learn the basic postures quickly and easily. Adding yoga into your daily life can be very simple as you can see it can only take minutes a day, you can start straight away and begin enjoying the many benefits.

The next step is to find the style of yoga that suits you best and to commit to a regular program. Your mind and body will thank you.

Finally, if you enjoyed this book, then I'd like to ask you for a favor, would you be kind enough to leave a review for this book on Amazon? It'd be greatly appreciated!

Further Reading

Article: "Yoga Poses for the Chakra System"

http://www.yogajournal.com/article/beginners/asanas-for-the-chakra-system/

General website: yoga.about.com

Article: "Meditation Tips for Beginners"

http://www.freemeditation.com/meditation-basics/meditation-tips-for-beginners/

.